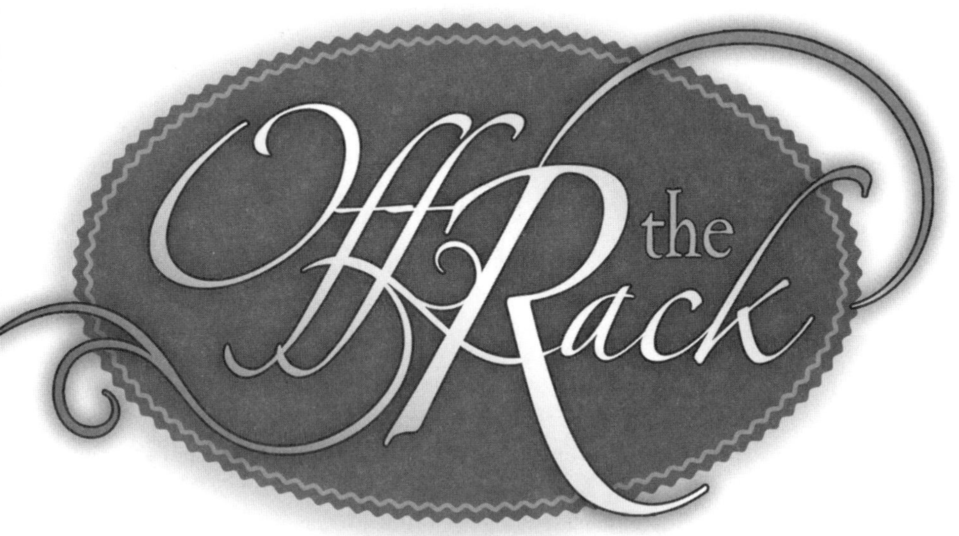

GENAE GIRARD

Strong Books ➤ Avon, Connecticut

OFF THE RACK

Strong Books
PO Box 715
Avon, CT 06001-0715
(800) 562-4357
www.OffTheRackBook.com

Disclaimer. This book is based on true events, but certain liberties have been taken with names, places, persons, organizations and dates for purposes of confidentiality. However, every effort has been made to present accurate information with regard to the author's personal experiences. Therefore, the author and publisher are not responsible for any unintentional resemblance to actual persons or organizations described in this book. No book, including this one, can replace the services of a qualified physician or other health-care professional. The author and publisher are not engaging in rendering medical or counseling services. If problems appear or persist, the reader should consult with a well-chosen physician, health-care or mental-health professional. Accordingly, the author and publisher expressly disclaim any liability, loss, damage or injury caused by the contents of this book.

Book design © TLC Graphics, www.TLCGraphics.com
Cover by: Tamara Dever; Interior by: Erin Stark

Printed in the United States of America.

ISBN: 978-1-928782-22-3

Thank you Bryant, Allison, Kevin, Matt, Erika,
my parents and all the young cancer survivors
that made this story possible.

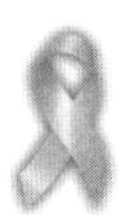

Table of Contents

Introduction

DIDN'T YOU KNOW? EVERYBODY'S DOING IT THESE DAYS… being diagnosed with cancer. Every day I see someone in the news publicly announcing their cancer diagnosis. It doesn't discriminate; it hits famous people, rich people, young and old. I never paid much attention to the fuzzy background reports I could vaguely hear on television. I was far removed from the idea of fighting cancer because I was young, vibrant and unaware. That changed abruptly with one visit to the doctor when time stood still. I was diagnosed with stage II breast cancer at age 36. I was divorced, dating, childless and desperate for information about experiences that people in my situation might have written. The bookshelves were barren of similar experiences. I found stories that were overly religious in tone and stories of sadness and depression that generally brought me down emotionally. I got through my initial treatment and grew from it exponentially. Using the tools of self-reflection, humor and a little backbone, I am here to tell you that you can get through it, and you are not alone.

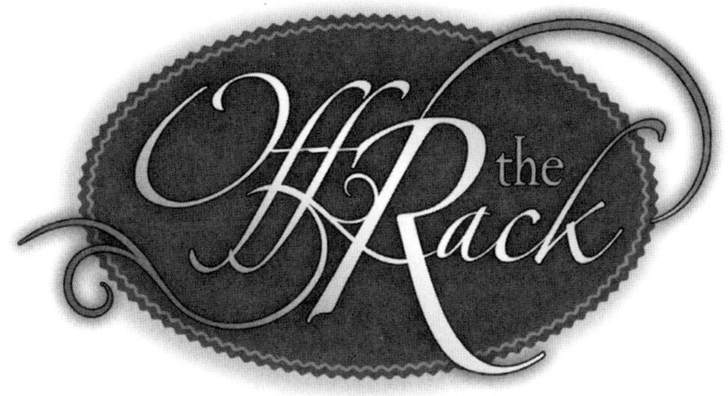

Chronicles of a Thirty Something, Single Cancer Survivor

THE DICTIONARY DEFINES CANCER AS:

A malignant tumor of potentially unlimited growth that expands locally by invasion and systemically by metastasis **b:** an abnormal bodily state marked by such tumors.

Did you catch the key word: invasion? Too many of us are being invaded against our will. I was invaded sometime before July of 2006 (the date of my diagnosis), and I am sure that I didn't request the presence of any cancer Martians to dock and set up shop in my breast. This news flash came across my life's radar screen completely and totally uninvited. I did, indeed, feel like I had been invaded. Throughout these pages are my observations and how I coped.

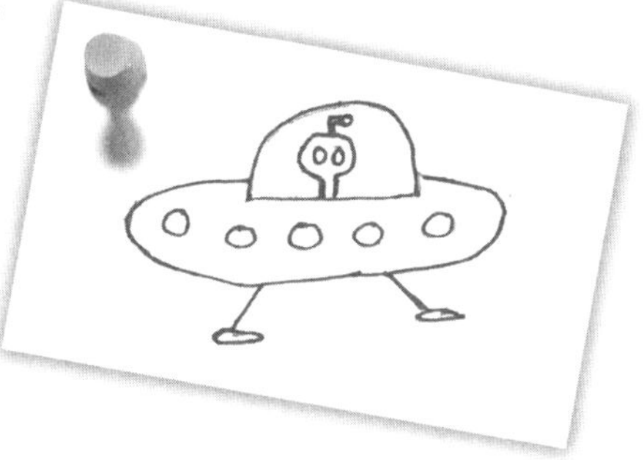

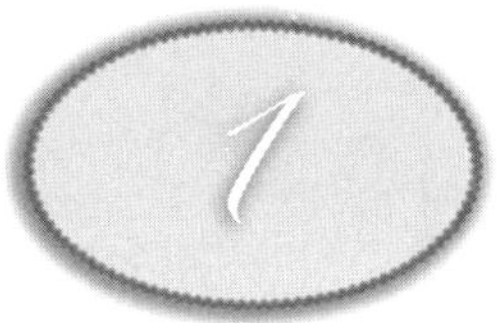

Poked, Prodded and Diagnosed

NOTHING CAN PREPARE YOU FOR THAT APPOINTMENT in which you find out you have been invaded by aliens (cancer). For me, my breast cancer diagnosis was reminiscent of the cartoon where Wile E. Coyote is forced off the canyon cliff by the Roadrunner.

My surgeon had just read my pathology report, and I could tell by his face that it wasn't good. "Well," he said, "your test came back positive for breast cancer." I burst out crying as he handed me a tissue. He was so kind and generous with information. I later wondered how many people he would have to inform about their invasions. I thought, *What a depressing message to have to deliver all day. That ranks right up there in occupational status with elephant cage cleaning and rat removal.*

I left the surgeon's office and fought to keep it together in the elevator as I donned my sunglasses to protect my fragile tear-filled eyes from the sun and onlookers' concern. I sat in my car in the parking lot for over ten minutes not able to grasp the concept of how a thirty-six year old that had never been to a doctor besides the yearly gynecologist appointment could now have a life threatening disease. After contemplating the ramifications of my situation, I began the wailing cry. This kind of cry is so loud that it projects from the diaphragm. It was a kind of cry that you would see on stage or in a movie: "Stella, Stella!" from a *Street Car Named Desire* comes to mind.

I transitioned from wailing to sobbing and started having feelings of "Woe is me" and thoughts of "Wow, I am dying." I couldn't fathom this… I own a company, I am an artist, I am a physically fit person and I love life. This completely sucks. I felt like Charlie Brown standing on the pitchers mound with the rain cloud only pouring down on me. As the fight or flight stress response kicked in, my heart beat faster, I started sweating and my gut wrenched with pain. Why had this invasion occurred in me? Had my body sent out signals to the invading aliens that I was ripe for the mother ship to come dock in my breast? Did I have exposure to too many chemicals in my childhood? Maybe I licked lead paint as a child when nobody was looking. I wanted answers.

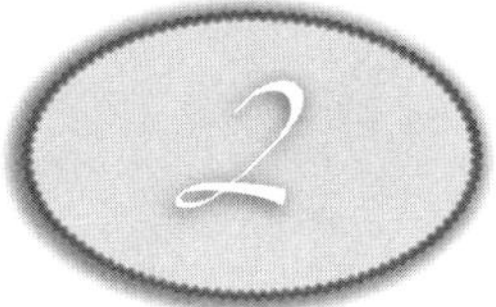

Fear

WHAT WAS IT ABOUT THIS DIAGNOSIS THAT MADE ME have gut wrenching fear? My mind raced to try and fill in the landscape of blanks that existed in my head. My mind was spinning like a rat running on an exercise wheel. There were too many questions and not enough answers. With my mind left to its own spinning devices I could not sleep or function as I had before. I now knew why people used the term "gripping" and "fear" in the same sentence. There was a lack of control as my alien invasion was rapidly dividing in my body. I felt like a "sitting duck."

I have read about fear existing in the unconscious mind. Over time it has served its purpose of extending our survival. I'm sure it came in handy while cavemen ran from predators. Herein lies the irony for me. I have a fear response to look both ways before I cross the street. I lock the front door for fear of burglars. I don't cross through dark alleys to potentially protect me from criminal intent. My fear response kicks in evolutionally to potentially protect my life, yet the fear of this cancer and lack of control could ultimately affect my existence.

I decided to try and conquer my fears by actually befriending them. This would entail recognizing the symptoms and becoming aware of their presence, and devoting my conscious mind to it. When I would start to feel the stress mechanisms of breathing harder, faster heartbeat, sleeplessness and irritability, I would acknowledge the symptoms and be aware. This self-dialog would eventually lead to a less stressful situation in which I could focus on the here and now vs. the "what ifs." The "what ifs" were the danger and could leave me drowning in fear.

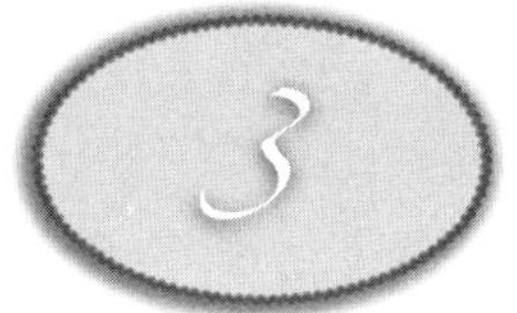

Inconvenience

After the sadness and shock dissipated, it occurred to me how very inconvenient this diagnosis was. When the treatment schedule was handed down to me I was horrified at how this protocol would eat away at more than a full year of my life. These aliens obviously forgot to check my schedule before setting up shop. Would I be able to work? Would the treatment work? Would my life be on hold? And there lies the kicker. There are no finite answers when it comes to cancer. I remember when I was a kid there was this movie called *Innerspace* where a man gets miniaturized along with a tiny spaceship and gets injected into another man. How cool would that be if I could miniaturize the Air Force's best pilot to go in and declare war on my cancer. It turns out—all science fiction aside—that our best lines of defense are surgery, chemotherapy and radiation. I had to ramp up my inner strength to get ready for battle without the help of the tiny soldier I dreamt about injecting.

Being a business owner, I have been trained in the art of researching. Researching started for me when I was a child. This was before the process became computerized. Surpassing all child labor laws, when my father was going through medical school, I would often accompany him to the library where I would get nickels and dimes to seek out dusty medical journals and articles. I would schlep them over to the copier and copy one page at a time. My nose would twitch as the dust clouds erupted from the pages. I enjoyed the exposure to the books. They were like pieces of history ripe for the picking. This process catapulted me into a deluge of reading and researching. I have always felt that if you are going to dive into unfamiliar territory, books and knowledge are the best way to build your wall of protection.

My family mostly sang the praises of the theme, "Pull Yourself Up By Your Bootstraps." As you read this book, you will more than likely see that theme raise its head to wink at you every now and then. Because of this bootstrap mentality, my brother and I were told to do things that most parents would consider surprising. Whether you liked it or not, it taught courage. Courage to be a doer, and to push your fear down and raise your confidence up.

After my cancer shock, I went to the bookstore and bought every book I could find pertaining to my diagnosis. I must have had about twenty balancing in my arms like the Leaning Tower of Pisa. I remember in college I was one of those people that had problems concentrating on reading and retaining. Something more interesting than the Kirkegaard I was reading always seemed to distract me. I could literally read a couple of pages, only to look up and realize that I hadn't remembered anything I just read. Maybe I was experiencing a new type of temporary Alzheimer's or a brain hiccup that causes you to lapse. This process completely changed when I got home from the cancer book trip to the bookstore.

I read every one of the books in less than three days. Fishing for answers pertaining to your health and existence tends to add urgency to the reading process. I started to feel like I was back in college researching information for a thesis, only this thesis was my life. I wanted to round out my research to include other women who had already gone through this. I called the Breast Cancer Resource Center in my area, which was a wealth of knowledge. They offered a breast cancer support group comprised of women under forty years of age. I had found women just like me. I was not alone in my fight to win over the alien invasion. I had a team. A team of like-minded individuals paddling in the same boat as I was.

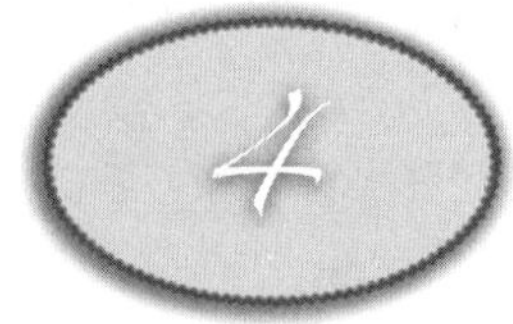

You Didn't Do Anything Wrong

My first visit to the oncologist was a fact-finding mission. Everything about the building itself was daunting. What is it about hospitals and clinics? They always have that smell. It is a sanitized sterility smell. It isn't foul, but it isn't pleasant either. If you were blindfolded you would immediately know that you were in a healthcare facility. Polished floors, industrial looking windows, corporate calendars from every major pharmaceutical company peeking back at you from every cubical. In the waiting area there was a collection of health magazines peering back at me, almost mocking me as if they knew of my diagnosis. "Read me, read me! And you can feel even worse about yourself!" The television in the waiting room was always tuned onto a news channel. The volume was always so low that you couldn't hear anything, and yet folks would stare glossy-eyed at the screen until their name was called.

Almost everyone in the waiting room was missing hair and looking weak. I was a first timer, and the crowd was well aware of that. I peered past the waiting room and saw multiple reclining chairs with people and their I.V. poles. I thought to myself, *That will soon be me.* Fear started to rear its ugly head and I breathed quietly and slowly to reach some level of calm.

I struck up a conversation with a lady sitting next to me. Strange, you tend to talk about anything and everything in this waiting room except for your diagnosis. It's almost as if you think that by talking about it you might catch what the other person has…or if you use denial, maybe the time spent in this place will seem as if we were never there. I have had similar experiences at the grocery store or during a casual discussion in the shopping mall.

As my name was called, I meandered my way down the long hallway to meet my nemesis, the scale. The scale was very industrial looking. It looked as if you could weigh a baby elephant or a UPS package on its base. My temperature was then recorded. The nurses who were multi-taskers could weigh you and take your temperature in your inner ear simultaneously. This wasn't the most pleasant experience, especially if you happened to be moving. Like the serving lady at the cafeteria reaching for the mashed potatoes with one hand and scooping up green beans with the other. They were pros and on a tight schedule.

I continued walking the Green Mile down the hallway to my oncologist's waiting room. *Typical,* I thought. Two chairs, one that rolls, one that is stationary and a patient exam table. On the wall was a collage of many of my oncologist's family vacation photos and everyone in them was grinning from ear to ear. There were pictures in Hawaii and other tropical locations as well as pictures of special events. I wondered about the psychology of this wall scrapbook. Was this an attempt to personify himself as a great guy so that I wouldn't feel animosity toward him as he prescribed my poisonous drip of chemotherapy drugs? Would his patients like him better knowing that his family looked like the great American dream? I was suspicious.

As I was sitting on the exam table making crinkling noises from my butt moving around on the table paper, my oncologist finally entered. He introduced himself and said, "First off, I want you to know that this isn't your fault." I was a little awestruck by that comment. I guess many patients come in wondering, *What did I do to myself to cause this alien invasion?* This statement seemed a little rehearsed to me, like, "Welcome to Mc Oncology, would you like to try our new Mc Treatment?" I looked at him and said, "I know that, doc, now let's get down to business."

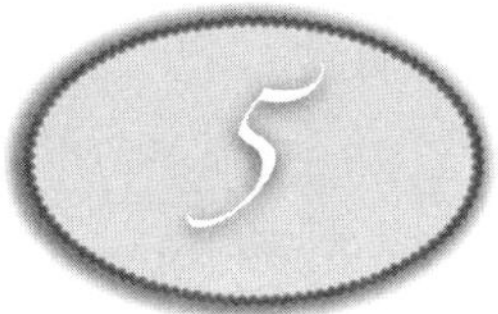

I'm Not a Sheep

MY FATHER IS A RADIOLOGIST AND WENT TO SCHOOL BACK in the 1960s. *He is going to kill me for disclosing that.* At that time, doctors were actually learning basic medicine and then moving into a specialty. Now, there is so much to learn in specialty fields and so little time that doctors spend very little time learning basic practices. God forbid that I am in a specialist's office and need CPR. I would be screwed. Most doctors have their own specialty, which doesn't trickle over into other fields. I found that this caused some problems for me, the patient. When I would speak to one doctor about a particular area of my diagnosis, they could only tell me about their particular area of specialty. Herein lies the problem. There is only one me, and every treatment whether it was surgery, chemotherapy or diagnostic reading, impacted this individual "me". Although all my doctors consulted and worked as a team, I decided I would have to become a specialist about my own diagnosis and body. I would have to research my situation, query others that have been in my situation and ask questions upon questions until I felt comfortable with my decisions.

My particular doctor trail looked something like this.

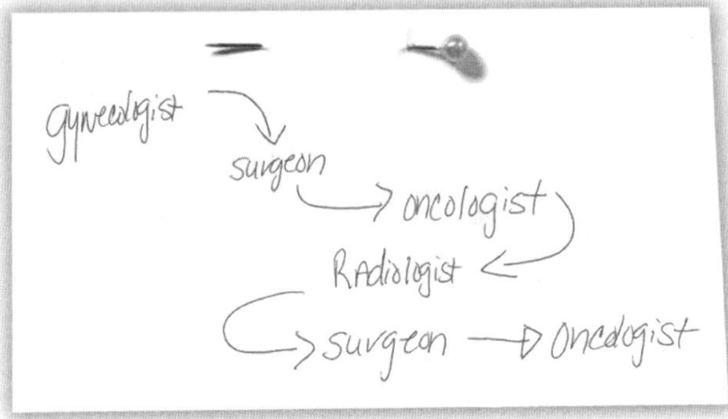

I would need to become knowledgeable in all the subjects pertaining to me in order to make an informed decision about my health care. If I didn't understand something, I would probe to dig further. We are all different; therefore, each treatment should be customized to fit our needs. Besides, not one of the doctors I was working with had ever been through such treatments themselves.

I was once sitting in the chemo chair and there was a woman who had just had her port surgically implanted. The nurses were trying to insert the needle in her port, but something was terribly wrong. You could see that she was in agony and immense pain. After a few tries, I said, "Stop! Something is wrong."

It definitely got the nurses' attention as they quit focusing on the task at hand, and rather focused on the fact that they were hurting the patient. As I sat in the chair that day, my overly creative brain started imagining medical training that required all of the chemo nurses and doctors to have to experience at least one dose of the chemo poison. I wondered how that would impact their level of knowledge and understanding. Maybe if staff members were intimately aware of the process, it only would have taken one scream from the patient with the new port to get reassessed. There is no substitute for first hand knowledge.

There is no substitute for filling out medical paperwork currently either. I remember that when I was healthy, filling out paperwork at the doctor's office was as easy as 1-2-3. All of the little boxes I checked were, "No". I was so healthy that I didn't pay much attention to the form. When I was diagnosed, all of a sudden I had to pay close attention to the form in front of me. The clipboard became my nemesis. Cancer? Yes. Weight gain? Yes. Night sweats? Yes. Pain? Yes. I came to the conclusion that I much preferred being the "No" patient rather than the "Yes" one, who, simultaneously, was now off the preferred insurance list.

The most important step I took was to take control of my treatments by educating myself on all aspects of treatment. I was prepared with questions before I talked to my doctors, and it made all the difference in the world. I went into the treatment protocol without a "one size fits all" mentality. It's my body and I only have one, was my thought. I am not a sheep, and I do not follow the masses. I am an individual and I am unique.

There were so many scientific changes during my treatment. New pharmaceuticals were being released, as were new treatment protocols and new equipment. It was tough to keep up with everything. I wanted to make sure that I wasn't missing any piece of my recovery puzzle. I remember in the beginning that I was overly concerned with other women's treatment protocols. I was concerned if someone was getting a certain drug over a certain period of time and I wasn't. Or if someone was getting radiation vs. what I was getting. It reminded me of standing in the registration line for college as a freshman. Many of the upper class students had an air of confidence as they collected registration papers and books and like seasoned professionals knew exactly where to go. I was in a panic not knowing where to go, what to do or who to see. I would watch and listen carefully, trying to figure out my strategy of how to navigate the campus. I didn't want to miss out on anything. Similarly, when I was diagnosed I would watch listen and try to figure out what my plan of navigation would be. It concerned me when someone was getting a different protocol than mine. As I made my way through this journey and started to become more relaxed, I realized that this was not a good thing. Everyone's diagnosis is different and therefore the treatments should be different. My fear mirrored the fact that I didn't want to miss out on anything that could prolong my life.

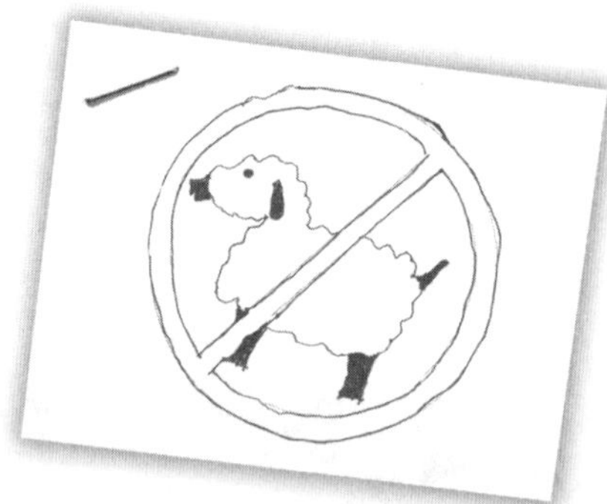

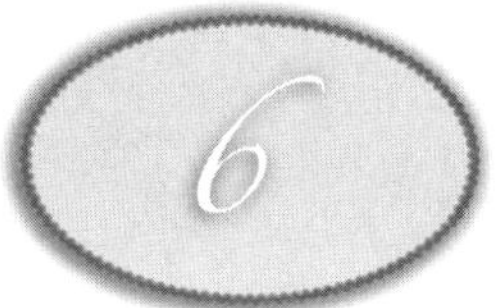

Expiration Date

I REMEMBER WHEN I WAS FIRST DIAGNOSED WITH BREAST cancer I was thrown into a whirlwind of statistics related to the type of tumor I had, and whether or not I was lymph node positive. All of these pieces of information were invaluable when determining the characteristics of my cancer and making treatment decisions. Medical professionals and the different cancer societies have compiled statistical data on all cancers based on treatment protocols that can give you an estimate for your chances of survival. *Wow, a mathematical formula that can guess my life span.* I dove into the world of statistics looking for answers. While treading water, I found that the statistics were useful in determining the best course of action for my treatment; however, I found the term "survival rate" to be cement shoes during the swim.

There are actual software programs that exist in which you can plug in your cancer statistics and based on your treatment protocols and nature of your cancer you can see what your chances of survival are in year increments. I chose not to input my statistics. I thought, *Why should I live my life knowing that a computer with a lightning fast processor just coughed up a statistical curve that determined my life expectancy. Maybe it would be easier if we were all born with an expiration date stamped on our ass. I think I will just live life playing by God's rules instead.*

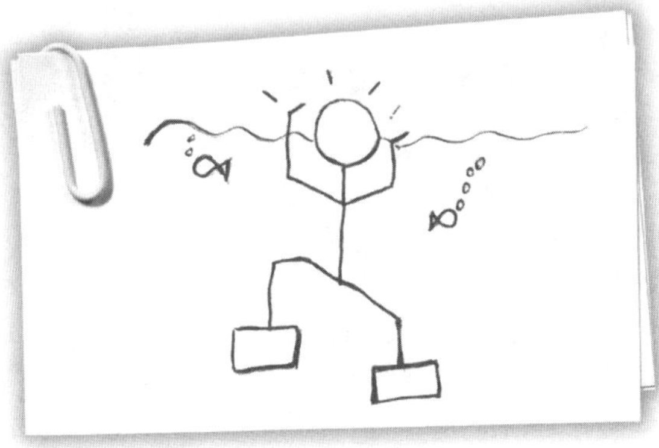

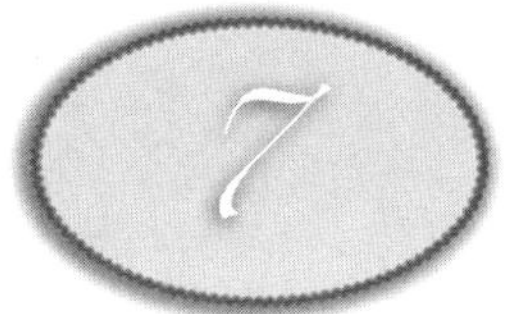

Death Becomes Us

I ATTENDED A CONFERENCE ONCE WHERE I HEARD A speaker who had a very aggressive form of breast cancer. She was young and beautiful. She was sitting smartly dressed on a stool addressing the audience. You wouldn't have realized that she was battling a disease, except for the blatant oxygen tank hooked up to her. Her theme revolved around the idea of everyone having a brand. She said the best way to find that brand is to write down your life stories and to look for common words and themes. When you do this, she said, your strengths and brand will appear.

I decided that after my diagnosis, I didn't want my brand to be cancer. My brand is Genae. Unique, quirky and with a little whipped cream on top. This speaker was someone special too. Although she was obviously straining to breathe, she still sat tall and confident as she addressed the crowd. As she began to speak, she told the story of a "Woe is me" moment where she was traveling by car and having extreme trouble breathing due to her illness. She called her accountant husband sobbing and said, "Jim, I am dying." He paused and said, "Yes, dear, we all are."

I contemplated hearing those words. Isn't that the truth? We all are in different degrees and stages of life, but that is the final outcome. It is not morbid for me to hear that, although some might find the concept too abrasive. I find it comforting. It allows me to relax and be in the moment. There is no rush to find meaning in life. I can just be. It took a man who crunches numbers for a living to break the concept down into something manageable. I saw the speaker with breast cancer long before I was diagnosed, but this pearl of wisdom has always stuck with me.

One reason this topic rings so true is that life is terminal. Again, as a business owner, I liked to reengineer this thought. Looking at my life span and how lucky I was to be brought into this world and not knowing when and where I would be taken seemed like a great ride. If everyone focused on when the Grim Reaper was going to rap at the door, what a dreary existence it would be. I am just like all the great beings in nature existing, growing and evolving. There is nothing to be more grateful for.

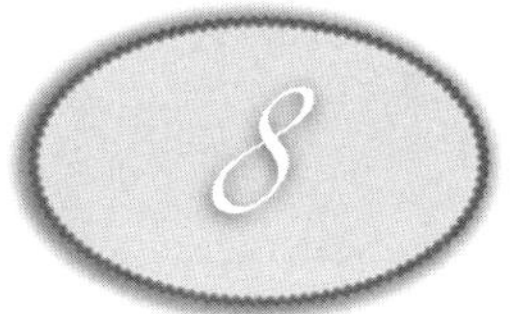

Arming Myself

WHEN YOU ARE FIRST DIAGNOSED WITH AN ALIEN INVASION you are in a state of shock and sometimes disbelief. I wasn't in the most stable frame of mind already in my life. My husband had an affair and we separated, plus I had stress from my business. This news was like I walked onto a land mine already having a flesh wound. I would have to reach deep. I moved from shock into full steam ahead on my treatment course. I have always considered myself a competitor, so being in pretty good health (other than the cancer) at age thirty-six, I decided I would get as aggressive as I could during my treatment. Chemotherapy was looming so I decided I would arm myself with acupuncture, meditation, and prayer and healing school. After all, I was going into the ring to fight the alien invasion and it was time to get some weapons in place.

I have to say that I wasn't a very cooperative acupuncture pincushion. The acupuncturist said, "Stick out your tongue; I need to examine it to see what your deficiencies are." I had cancer, for God's sake. Does that count as a deficiency? If I opened my mouth would there be an alien ship waving back at her saying, "Hi, we have set up shop and are alive and well." Being somewhat influenced by Western medical traditions, as well as coming from a technical radiologist dad in the family, I uttered, "Um, can you just stick some needles in me and we'll call it good?"

Prayer and healing school gave me a lot of reflection. I went over scripture and had small focus groups that prayed over me. I was supposed to close my eyes and think about the cancer leaving my body. True to form, I opened my eyes and peeked. I was amazed at the outpouring of emotion everyone in my group expressed toward me. Some were crying, some were speaking a different language all together. Some were laughing the cancer out of my body. They prayed for my peace, and peace is what I received.

Meditation was a tougher nut to crack. People like me, who are "Type-A", don't sit still and remove all of those thoughts flowing through their brain. People like me are thinkers. If I felt the stress entering my body I knew that I would have to get a grip on this demon before it caused more damage. Stress of the unknown during your treatment is almost impossible to avoid. Every turn is like pulling the handle on a Vegas slot machine; you are never quite sure what it is you are going to roll. As I practiced and became better at it, the process became easier. It took coaching over about two years to help me gradually work it out. I became more mindful of living in the present. It seems like certain personality types are more prone to success in meditation, but once you start practicing, your whole outlook changes and you become more peaceful. Getting there is the tough part.

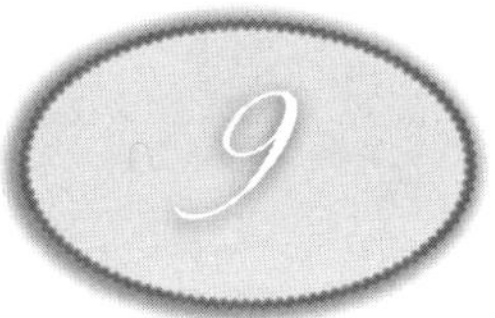

Bridge of Friends both Human and Furry

Having people around me that had experienced cancer was invaluable. It is an exclusive club that can share important information, good and bad, and that understands where you are coming from. They help you to make informed decisions along the way as well as marvel at the fact your stubbly hair is growing back after chemo. I joined a local group of women under forty that were all facing similar issues. Most of these women had different issues than the older ones diagnosed. Mainly these issues revolved around fertility. I was concerned that when I first went to the meetings it would be like the twelve step program for cancer survivors. "Hello, my name is Genae and I am a cancer survivor." "Hello, Genae." Thank God it wasn't like that at all. The women in this group were on a different life maturity plane. There was also a level of respect that you might find at an officer's club or veterans group. It was a great bunch of women that were all in the same boat. When I started talking to other survivors about our medical procedures, a medical foreign language unfolded. Put a veteran group of survivors in with a group of civilians and see how long before the head scratching and looks of confusion begin. These were women warriors.

There were some women I met along this journey that chose not to communicate with friends outside their circles. I once met a girl that was going through chemo at the same time I was. She was a little younger and recently married. Her husband would come with her to chemo treatments and wait with her. I hit it off with her and thought that she would be a great person to know outside of this poisonous realm. I reached out to her via phone and email but there was no reciprocation. I have met a few people along the way that keep their diagnosis very close. Too close. When you are first diagnosed the rainbow range of emotions and thoughts that plow through your brain is vast. For me it was like a great trauma I experienced that I needed to talk about just as a hurricane victim or a war veteran. The more I talked and discussed the trauma with like-minded survivors, the more the fear and pain were relieved.

My two Labradors relieved the pain as well. When I felt like hell and had just been pumped full of my chemotherapy poison, they would jump up right next to me on the couch and sniff me. I must have smelled like poison too. They would sniff my skin and ear and then proceed to lie down, head in my lap. It always amazed me how much they seemed to know. I am definitely a dog person.

I once was on the way to an outdoor concert with one of my Labs. I was with my boyfriend and his two children. We decided that we were hungry and wanted to go to a Mexican restaurant nearby. What were we going to do with the dog? I told my boyfriend's son in his wise old eight years of age to grab my Lab's leash and don my dark sunglasses and pretend to be blind. I then asked the wait staff if it was okay for us to bring the dog through the hallway and outside on the patio. They agreed. Meanwhile, my boyfriend's son is holding onto the leash, eyes shielded by sunglasses while my lab is chewing table scraps from the floor as we walk. This furry vacuum cleaner was blowing our cover. She did get a grilled chicken breast out of it.

I dreamed of taking one of my Labs into the chemotherapy ward with me. I thought about pretending that she was a service dog so that she could keep me company while I was getting juiced. Somehow at the first sign of a cookie or someone snacking, I could see her flying down the hall getting tangled in everyone's I.V. lines. Maybe she would try to bite a nurse for trying to inject me. On second thought, it probably wasn't a good idea.

No Sympathy Please

I GATHERED PRETTY QUICKLY THAT MOST PEOPLE DON'T KNOW what to say when you are diagnosed. When I would tell a friend there would be a brief uncomfortable pause before they responded. "I'm sorry" is one of the more traditional responses. Followed by "Holy Shit" and a side of "Are you kidding me?" Really, the last response I wanted was sympathy. I guess as a patient you don't even know how to respond to your own diagnosis, so how are innocent bystanders supposed to respond?

I have discussed with people what the correct response might be… .I have determined that there is no correct answer. While going through treatment, the most powerful bystanders were the ones that just listened. People offering to help out when I was tired or keep me up-beat made all the difference in the world. I felt like I was grasping for some sense of normalcy. During the treatment I lost almost all sense of normalcy. My appearance was different, my energy levels were different, I was different. Hard to admit though when you have never been ill before. I had always depended on myself. This was a life lesson I would soon become more familiar with; you can't always go it alone.

Laughing was important to my sanity as well. I focused on trying to get in at least one good belly laugh a day. Day to day stories of my friends going through treatment and what they encountered kept me rolling in the aisles. A good friend of mine was in my support group and going through cancer treatments. She had a great sense of humor and actually had to go through chemo during a pregnancy. Talk about a woman warrior. I met her first at a support group meeting and she was about 7 months pregnant. Many people asked her at the time about why she had started wearing a wig. She said she was tired of the "double sympathy stare." People would look at her pregnant belly, then up at her bald head, and give that sympathy look that we all hated.

My overly hilarious pregnant friend's husband's response was a little unorthodox when she was diagnosed. She looked at him and said, "Honey, will you still love me after a double mastectomy and breast implants?" He responded by saying, "Oh honey, you know I am not a breast man. I am more of a butt man. Now if you had ass cancer, that would be a different story." One good chuckle is like a spoonful of medicine that eventually quiets the mind and relaxes the anxiety that cancer patients face.

The truth is, I didn't want people feeling sorry for me during my treatment. Because of my appearance, I couldn't always hide my treatment and the stares I received were plentiful. Empathy would have been better. Don't get me wrong. Sometimes the slightest bit of sympathy is worth something. For example, going through treatment allowed me to get an upgrade at a hotel in Cozumel, Mexico. After one glance from the hotel clerk looking at my bandana covered head, I was pushed to the Lido rooms facing the ocean. Not bad for a freshman patient. Besides, have you ever tried to wear a wig in island humidity?

Fertility Instability

WHILE CONDUCTING MY CHEMOTHERAPY RESEARCH, I learned that I might never be able to have children. Chemo would have close to a 50/50 shot at rendering me infertile. *Not good odds,* I thought. I could do a hormone free egg sparing procedure that may or may not protect the eggs. I was thirty-six and not married, but I appreciated the choices that were presented to me. The idea of having a child was tough. I was recently divorced and getting closer to forty. This created anxiety pressure and fear aside from my cancer diagnosis.

I remember exactly where I was when my older brother called to tell me he and his wife were pregnant. I was standing in the frozen foods aisle of the grocery store comparing pre-packaged diet meals. I was so excited to have a niece or nephew…but selfishly a sense of panic came over me. Being an overachiever has its downfalls. Would I be missing out on one of life's biggest joys? Would I have regrets? Did I need to find a husband pronto? Maybe the fear stemmed from knowing that naturally the whole family's focus shifts to grandchildren rather than adults. At some point the adults are like 5-day-old potato salad that no one wants to partake of but no one wants to throw away. And then there is the cease and desist of Christmas gifts. I knew what was around the corner. It's a natural occurrence for the ebb and flow to move to the younger kiddos. Through a couple of years of psychotherapy I had gained many of the tools that I needed to self reflect and work through these life questions. I decided that I would take a step back and just let things unfold.

I hadn't been someone who was insistent on having kids. Some people might find that unfathomable. I do find that children in your life are a blessing. Watching the discovery process is my most favorite time. The cognitive process not fully developed is a hoot to watch. Within the uncertain possibilities of having children, I realized quickly that I wasn't prepared for the effects that chemo was going to have on my body. Being menopausal at age 36 is like a thermostat in your body just smoked crack cocaine. Most nights I would lay awake sweating like I was completely combustible from the inside out. Most women going through the change have a slow drop in estrogen that allows them to transition into menopause. Not me. Chemo kicked out the legs from my estrogen chair and left me on fire. What happens to a woman when you take away her hair, boobs, and hormones? Nothing good. I feel at least 10 years older. Before treatment I felt young and spry, but now my joints have started creaking, I have deeper lines in my face, kind of like my leather couch. My chemotherapy brain is getting forgetful; is this the beginning of Alzheimer's? My mastectomy surgery and rebuilt boobs ache, and the skin on my hands looks 50 years old. Night sweats? What the hell is that about? "I'm on fire! I'm on fire! Put me out! Put me out! No wait! I'm cold, I'm cold!" I wake up in sheets that look like an Olympic swimmer just used them to towel off after a 100-meter race. What I am beginning to understand finally is that I have a new normal. I will never be or feel the same. I just needed to adjust my baseline.

How to Make the Most of the Drano Drip

THE FIRST DAY OF CHEMO I DIDN'T KNOW WHAT TO expect exactly. Fear might be a good word to describe it. I walked into a room with many people hooked up to I.V. pumps. The diversity of who was in the room was shocking to me. All races and ages were represented. I had now entered an exclusive club. Folks that were all ready hooked up to the I.V.s politely smiled and seemed to know that I was a chemo virgin. I had not yet been ravaged by the effects of the chemo chemicals. My boyfriend had come with me, insistent on being there while I went through the long drip process. They first pumped me full of a steroid and then with Adryomycin, which I nicknamed "the red dragon." We sat and joked and made the best of a life-changing situation.

During chemo you become painfully aware of weight gain and weight loss. I equate the weigh-in to the Heavy Weight Champion of the World or jockeys getting ready for the Kentucky Derby. Your weight determines how much Drano they need to juice you with and is therefore extremely important during every visit. Funny, when I think about it, weight has always been taboo in the sisterhood. It ranks up there with publicly announcing your age. There is another area that used to be taboo…showing your body. I used to be a prude. I dreaded going to the gynecologist and having to disrobe and don a paper gown. Boy has my outlook changed. After the fiftieth time of a doctor feeling and peering at your breasts you become so desensitized it's like the naked comfortable porn star waiting for the director to yell, "Action!"

I remember one of my most uncomfortable interactions with nakedness during a vacation to Jamaica. I was visiting a resort in Jamaica with a "Clothing Optional" island that you had to travel to by boat. My naiveté told me that "clothing optional" meant exactly that. When I took the boat over to the island I noticed that there was nothing "Clothing Optional" about it. There was a naked bartender, a naked dockhand and naked people drinking fru fru drinks in a community pool bar. It should have been illegal for these gravity challenged folks to publicly be out in their birthday suits. My prudish self took the ferry back to the mainland, bathing suit still intact.

After a year of treatments, the thought of donning a paper gown (open in the front) seems downright laughable. For a seasoned veteran like me, a quick, "hello" from a doctor or nurse was all I needed to break the ice. Actually, I have been trying to think of alternative uses for the ¼ oz. paper cape that could really make a difference in someone's life.

Pirate vest for children's play

Ground cover for picnic

When worn open to the back, bib for eating spaghetti

When wadded up, fire starter for barbecue.

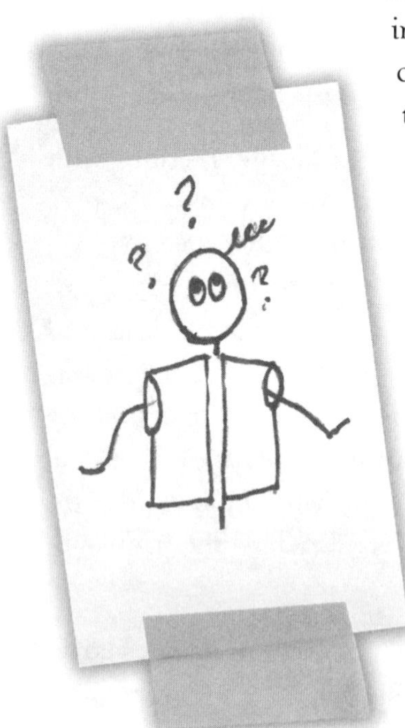

I have met the most interesting people in my life during chemotherapy. I met one woman that spends half of her time in Jamaica at a house she owns and half in the states where her husband teaches at a university. She was an experienced veteran and this was her second time going through chemotherapy. I struck up a conversation with her about the cancer experience she had endured. In the coolest Jamaican accent she said, "This shit isn't going to kill me. I'm not sure what will, but it isn't going to be breast cancer." You can't buy a better attitude anywhere.

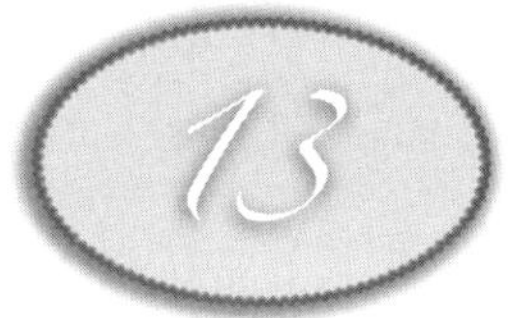

Journal Entry During Chemo

YOU CAN'T PREPARE YOURSELF FOR THE CHEMO ROOM experience. Everyone is there for the same reason: having toxic chemicals pumped into them to kill rapidly dividing cells. It is an exclusive club. There is no judgment in this room. It is void of discrimination. In the beginning of my treatment I couldn't get comfortable there, even though I was provided with a large chair that reclines about as far back as the astronauts sit while they are shot into space on board the space shuttle. I didn't want to be comfortable there. After six months of treatment I was comfortably numb about being there. This was the only other place besides prison where the words, "What are you in for?" resonated through the aisles.

Keeping a journal helps. On the day I'm writing this, I have been on chemo for one hundred and seventy one days. Who is counting? Me. The chemo room was recently expanded and rebuilt. They can put in double the number of patients in the new room and yet the chairs are totally full. I noticed that they have installed a small bell on the wall with a plaque. I have one more week before I get to ring a tiny bell on the wall that signifies my last treatment. I have watched others ring the bell and small eruptions of light clapping occur....not standing ovations. I am torn. Although I am ecstatic about the possibility of my Drano drip being over, I have great respect for others whose drip will never be dry. So I think I will forgo the small ringing of the bell out of respect for those not as lucky...besides, an air horn is more my style.

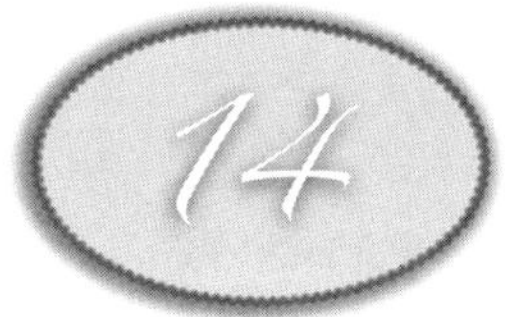

Wigging Out

AFTER TALKING WITH MY SUPPORT GROUP AND KNOWING that I would lose my hair in about 21 days depending on how hard the wind was blowing, I decided to go wig shopping. I was informed that consulting experts would be the best approach. I didn't want to resemble one of those bad damsels in distress characters in the movies wearing overly blonde wigs, a trench coat and sunglasses that cover up half of her face. They reminded me of the sixties when women used to block out the sun with oversized black sunglasses while all pumped up on valium.

The wig shop I found was also a full service salon. At that time I still had my hair but my chrome dome was imminent. I took a friend to help me choose a mane that didn't make me look like a hooker or Cousin It from the Adam's Family. As we entered the shop, many of the women turned and looked at me. It was if I had spinach stuck between my teeth or ketchup on my shirt. I could tell that they had a pretty good grasp on why I was there.

One of the women in the shop told me to come sit down at her station. She immediately chose a color and style that was similar to my own. The stylist put a cap on me, then put the wig on my head. As I was sitting with the wig on, low and behold my friend cruised right by me. *Hmmm*, I thought, *this could have a fun incognito quality about it. I could become someone else in the blink of an eye with the tug of a wig.* Six hundred dollars later, my wig came home with me.

My wig was human hair. I often wondered about the person or persons that donated the hair. I doubt they got any piece of the profits. My wig's name was Matilda. I named her that because when I was younger I thought only old people bought wigs and that was the oldest sounding name I could conjure up. My wig was hot and itchy but easy to style. When I was finished sporting Matilda I would let her sleep on a Styrofoam head with metal pins that held her on straight. If I placed the pins just right, they resembled Frankenstein bolts sticking out of the head. I had the wig on the bathroom counter, and every once in a while I would freak myself out by flicking the bathroom light on and seeing the Styrofoam head staring back at me. For a second, I would panic, not remembering she was there. Maybe I have watched too many horror movies and need to switch to a different genre.

Mane Loss

I WAS CONFIDENT THAT I WOULD LOSE MY HAIR DURING chemotherapy. Most of the women in my support group said, "Expect your hair to fall out about 21 days after starting treatment." The mane countdown had begun. I had no concept of what I was going to look like without hair. I wasn't even sure if my head was completely round. I thought it was because I looked at my baby pictures when I had barely any hair. It appeared to be round, but rather large. For much of my infant life I looked like I had a comb-over. The kind of hair all brushed over to the top to resemble more hair than what you actually have. The hair that when it is out of place your mother can apply a little spit to her fingers and slick it down. This was the only image I had of myself with very little hair. What is it about our society that reiterates that a woman's hair is her "Crown of Glory"? Well, I knew I was about to be dethroned.

When I was close to reaching my 21 days, I went to a party for one of the survivors in my support group. Her friends were throwing a party for her in which they had created a tubing float trip on a local river here in Texas entitled, "Thanks for the Mammaries." I was at the dinner party and my survivor friend said, "Wow! You still have your hair?" It was exactly 22 days after I had started my treatment. I told her that I knew I was doomed any day and laughed off the uncomfortable thought.

I had on a halter style top that night, which only had half of a back to it. As we all rose to toast my friend being finished with her treatment I could feel strands of hair sliding down my back as if on a slick spine rollercoaster. *Oh shit,* I thought....*this is it.* I spent the rest of the night keeping a smile on my face and not acknowledging the strands sticking to my shirt. When I would enter the restroom I looked in the mirror and saw more sable strands sticking like Velcro to my black shirt. I knew the more I messed with my hair, the more it would fall out so I purposely tried to keep my head straight. I knew the next day would be the dawning of a new day and the donning of clippers.

My boyfriend is an Army veteran, and I watched him confidently walk outside sporting clippers in his right hand. You could tell he had completed this process before and had no fear. I have a funny feeling that boot camp can do a lot of funny things to your head... literally. We had wine. A lot of wine, as we began the process of trimming and hedging our heads. We accomplished the task together. We sat back and looked at each other. I said to him, "You don't look so bad." "Well, thank you," he said, "neither do you." My head was immediately cold. It tingled and when the wind blew, it felt like someone had put menthol on my scalp. It felt strange to the touch, like low grit sandpaper. When I was completely finished, he gathered up the tufts of hair and balanced them on the top of my head. "You look like Elvis," he claimed. I really did.

After my hair was gone, I attended a support group meeting in which we could mentor other survivors that were just being diagnosed. I had my scarf on and situated myself at a U-shaped table that they had set up for us. Most of the group I had met before. As members in various stages of treatment made their way into the room, I took my scarf off to show a few people the fuzzy stage of my head. At the time, a pop music star, Britney Spears, had shaved her head and been seen in public without her golden strands. True to form, one of the young survivors said to me, "Hey, I will pay you to walk around the mall with me wearing a shirt that reads, 'I'm Britney's biggest fan.'" The room erupted with laughter. I left my scarf off all day.

Don't Underestimate the Importance of Denial

THE BEST WAY FOR ME TO SHARE THIS CONCEPT IS TO FIRST read a journal entry written while I was going through chemotherapy.

Journal Entry:

~Ode to Denial~

Webster defines **denial** as:

"a psychological defense mechanism in which confrontation with a personal problem or with reality is avoided by denying the existence of the problem or reality."

Every morning it's the same thing. I glance into the mirror and the sleepiness falls away from my brain and I am perplexed by the fuzzy head staring back at me. "Oh yes," I say to myself, "I forgot that I have cancer." I begin to gather up products that mask my appearance of going through chemo. My wig, my concealer, my eyebrow pencil.… I begin my routine of painting, wig straightening and globbing on various make up products in an effort to look like Cindy Crawford. I know I have gone too far when I see Tammy Faye Baker staring back at me in the mirror. When I have an appearance of normalcy I set out into the world without anyone being the wiser.

I have studied statistics. I have an extensive breast cancer library. I have interviewed doctors as well as many survivors. I feel like I have been in control and satisfied with my decisions thusfar. I have recently decided that on a day-to-day basis, I really appreciate denial.

You usually hear about denial in a negative connotation. I would like to portray it in a different light. Denial gives me a brain break. I can forget that every Friday I get juiced with Taxol. I can forget the fact that I have seven more treatments to go. I can forget that I filled in my eyebrows crooked yesterday so that I looked angry all day. I can forget for the last five months my shaved head has resembled David Carradine in the TV series *Kung Fu*.

So I would like to personally thank you, denial, for allowing me to forget for at least awhile that I am a breast cancer survivor. Thank you for the countless times you have helped me get through the day feeling great. Denial isn't just for psychology patients and desperate housewives anymore.

got denial?

Denial is a useful tool in my toolbox. It is like a screwdriver or any other major tool that you would use. In this case it is a tool for the mind. Dwelling on the fact I had cancer didn't seem very useful to me. It would zap my energy levels down low like the way a remote control toy zaps batteries. Dwelling on it would make my stomach get tight. That feeling of pain and nausea returned. Depression would take over and my fear and anxiety levels would rise. I didn't overuse denial. If I were to overuse denial, the tool would become dull, ineffective or even dangerous. I wasn't foolish. I kept up with all of my appointments, research, and questions for the doctors. If you were to ask me if I was sick, however, there was a good chance my denial voice would say, "Uh, no."

Off the Rack

IN THE BEGINNING I WASN'T SURE THAT I WOULD HAVE TO lose my boobs. Boobs? Isn't it amazing in America how many slang terms we use for breasts? I have heard more words used to describe breasts than those from a secret boys club. Rack, fun bags, jugs, hooters...just to name a few. A few years ago I may have found most of them derogatory. However, desensitization kicked in when I was getting ready to lose them.

After my lumpectomy, it became apparent that having a mastectomy would more than likely be the path I needed to take. I found out that I had won the genetic lottery by testing positive for the BRAC 2 gene. This means I am carrying the genetic mutation that increases the likelihood of the cancer developing in my breasts and ovaries. Ironically, I had never won anything until now. My inner alien was predisposed to setting up shop. It was like the campfire had already been started, where he could warm his feet by the fire and roast marshmallows.

The fear associated with surgery and the doctors removing my breasts was inconceivable. I had never had anything remotely wrong with me. I had never had surgery or even broken a bone. Here is where common sense started fighting with my ego. I started feeling like a Freud poster child. My common sense was telling me, "You need to get the cancer out of you. You need to protect the rest of the herd (body). You need to get both breasts taken out because of your genetic status. You need to prolong your life. Then my ego kicked in with, "Will I be disfigured? Will I ever be attractive enough to get married again? Will my Franken-boobs scare my boyfriend away?" After the voices in my head died down, there was one voice that shouted above the others. "You need to prolong your life, because, let's face it, you aren't done yet. You have things to do and people to see and you should make it count."

It's a weird thing, this surgical fear. It requires trusting a person or persons to cut you open and remove tissue, then put things back into you all with the purpose to save your life and make the final result look good. I was like a human canvas, but protecting the herd was the most important issue to me.

I found it surreal going to the plastic surgeon's office. There were women sitting in there for voluntary augmentation of boobs, thighs and nasal passages. Maybe there should be a special section....a front row if you will....for people going through cancer. Maybe we should be offered fresh baked cookies or receive a gold star of courage so that everyone knows that cancer chose us. This office was much different than my oncology office, with its high ceilings, large paintings and plush furniture all paid for by the reconstruction junction.

The procedure encompassed one surgeon taking out the breast tissue while a different surgeon put in the contraptions called expanders. Expanders are a temporary implant designed to inflate your skin over a period of four to six months in order to make room for your final implants. This concept originally perplexed me as I got a mental image of someone physically blowing up my chest like bubble gum, thus resembling Malibu Barbie.

There is a great indignity to losing body parts. I know as a woman I was pretty okay with my boobs. They weren't huge and they weren't tiny, they were like the last porridge bowl in the three bears.... "just right." I was divorced and had been dating a guy three months prior to my diagnosis. Losing boobs seemed to me to be a pretty major mountain to climb in a relationship, or maybe a major mountain to lose. I mean....how could a man find me attractive without them?

I went into the surgical facility and waited to be called. My boyfriend sat with me while we made small talk and read the newspaper. Everyone was glancing at everyone else. I know I was wondering what procedure they were there to receive. I think they were wondering the same thing. I would look up from the newspaper and they would immediately move their eyes in a downward fashion. The nurse called my name as I made my way through the halls. They smelled of coffee and sterility. As we made small talk with the nurse we made our way into an area with a large curtain hanging around a bed. I was asked to disrobe, put on the hospital gown and lay on the gurney style bed. It was time to say good-bye to my boobs and hello to the expanders that would be implanted in my chest.

The recovery facility was about as posh as a mid-grade hotel. Probably attributed to the fact that most of the procedures there are of a "pay up front" plastic surgery nature. I was out of surgery in just under six hours. They carefully removed the tissue on both sides and added my deflated saline expanders. I was coherent and moving around right afterwards. I knew what to expect. When I peeled down the surgical bra they put me in I had my two Frankenstein style incisions going across each mound. I had little or no bruising. It was surreal, but I wasn't shocked or surprised. I had been over this in my mind, realizing that this procedure would get the cancer out of me, thus allowing me the best chance to be rid of the aliens.

Setbacks

IT WAS TWO WEEKS AFTER MY EXPANDER SURGERY AND I went for a walk in my neighborhood. There is a hill I always climb and love getting to the top of it because one of my neighbors has a plastic goose she dresses up in different outfits depending on the time of year. This particular climb was no exception. As I reached the summit, there was the goose wearing a smart golf outfit with tweed knickers and an argyle vest. Her seamstress skills never disappoint.

As I began to make my trek back to the house I started feeling strange. Entering my house a feeling like hypothermia took over me. Strange thing was....it was about 89 degrees outside. I started shaking. It was the weirdest feeling. I knew something was not right. I hopped into the shower and tried to get my body temperature regulated. After one night of 104-degree fever, I decided to go to the doctor and they admitted me immediately to the hospital. Everyone I encountered said, "You may or may not have to get the expanders removed. After three days of waiting, it was determined that I had a MERSA infection, a type of staph infection that colonizes around implants and expanders.

Of my own accord, I took control of my infection and went to an infectious disease specialist. There were chairs lining the walls and they were completely filled. I was reading a book but slowly lifted my head only slightly to glance up at everyone in those chairs. My imagination went wild as I wondered what diseases everyone else had in that incubator of a room. I peered up and there was a picture of a smoking cowboy on the wall.

I got in to see the specialist and the first thing I said to him after introducing myself was, "You do realize you have a picture of a smoking cowboy on your clinic walls. That's a little ironic, don't you think? The doctor laughed and said, "Yes, I get that a lot."

After the doctor examined me, he said, "It doesn't look good. If you were my wife, I would recommend removing the expanders and waiting six months before trying the surgery again." This is not the first time I have heard the "wife" statement. I wonder if they teach that phrase somewhere in medical school? Or maybe it was on one of the various television hospital shows and doctors thought, *Hey, that's pretty good.* 1) Depicts the severity of the situation 2) Shows compassion as if you were a member of the family 3) Kind and endearing. It didn't really matter what the doctor said....all I could hear after "You will have to get the expanders out" was blah blah blah blah.

Shit, another blow. Although above the belt, this blow challenged the spirit that I had been maintaining through all of my surgical procedures. I would have to find some reserve still untapped. An aquifer of courage and strength needed to be drilled and accessed.

I was perplexed after my infection how a surgery to take the expanders out could be so fast. It took about an hour and a half and I was out the same day. I had bandages on and could feel the suture in my chest tightening. I would have to wait six months to try again with the expanders. I remember as I was driving home I looked down and could see that my bandaged chest resembled that of a twelve-year-old boy. As I drove home, my overactive mind started playing possibilities in my head. I started wondering if I happened to get home and my boyfriend was repulsed if I could potentially learn to be alone the rest of my life or even become a lesbian. I decided that I would just have to chance it and return to my life to see how others would respond.

To overcome the MERSA infection they would have to insert a PICC line into my arm, which is a tiny tube that goes up into your vein and into your body. I would have to inject myself for one hour every morning and every night with an intravenous antibiotic. This process would take more than four weeks. I felt like my life was dictated by this small plastic I.V. bag. It had control over my schedule. What pissed me off was that I had to sit still at home for one hour in the morning and one hour at night. Maybe I should really milk it and wear a hospital gown open in the back. During my four-week intravenous period I went to a party with my boyfriend one evening during this process. We were amongst many strangers. I had my PICC line bandage on with the port showing. I believe that many of the partygoers had partaken of something in a smokeable, illegal form.

One of the female smokers came up to me, eyes red, and asked, "What is that in your arm?"

"What?" I asked. "You mean you don't have one? Everybody is doing it."

"Oh, really?" she exclaimed, as she started to look worried.

Sometimes it is just too easy to mess with people.

The New Girls

SIX MONTHS AFTER THE MERSA INFECTION CLEARED UP I was ready to try getting the expanders put in again. The recommendation to get more blood flow to the site as well as more tissue to work with resulted in a Dorsi Latissimus Flap procedure. Isn't it funny how so many surgical procedures sound like Greek Philosophers? The surgery included pulling a muscle on either side of my back around to the front, then inserting the expander into the area. I would eventually be a human pretzel.

Six months after the second set of expanders were put in, I was ready for the swap out of the expanders to silicone implants. The scenario was all too familiar. I was in the waiting room and a nurse walked in to make sure I was in a gown and ready for the procedure. After six months of saline expansion I was right at 395 ccs.

The nurse asked me, "Okay, where are you now as far as your expansion? After I told her, she said, "Okay, I will bring in smaller, the same and larger sizes into the surgery room. *Hmmm*, I thought to myself, *I wonder what that means?* As the surgeon came in I got the proverbial surgical marker "road map" all over me dictating where the incisions and implants would be inserted. "Any questions?" the surgeon asked. "Yes, I do have one. Can I go bigger?" "Yes," he said, "we can go a little bigger, if you like." I responded, "Well, if we are gonna do this, let's do it bigger."

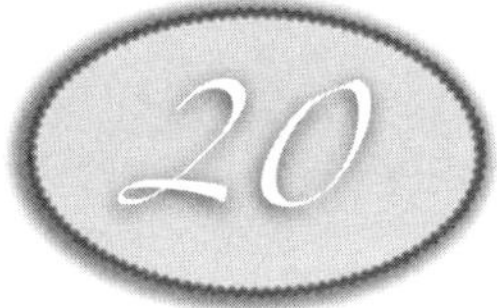

Gaining Pain

I HAD FINALLY PASSED THROUGH ALL OF MY SURGERIES, LIKE finally graduating from college. I had road maps of scars all over me. I later bought a t-shirt that said, "Scars are like tattoos only with better stories." I had never felt pain like this before. It would sneak up on me like a child playing hide 'n seek peering into the closet only to find and tag me. Sometimes when I wake up it grabs me by the back and tightens its grip on me as if to say, "Good morning." Sometimes it tricks me. When I am going about my everyday chores and feeling great, all of a sudden I stop in my tracks unable to move.

When you start taking things out of your body, adding some, and moving some around, there is bound to be some internal confusion. Why is it that pain has this way of taking control of your mind? It can alter your mood in a heartbeat. It can twist you into a bitch knot that you didn't tie. Then there is also the pain of fear. Fear can grip you and pierce your soul. It can take over if you aren't careful. There is one thing I have learned about pain. It lets me know I'm alive. It lets me know that I am capable of feeling life. So pain and I will learn to co-exist, but pain will not be in control of this mother ship.

Mirror Mirror on the Wall

I USED TO HAVE A GREAT RELATIONSHIP WITH MY BATHroom mirror. Let's just call it "Amir". I could casually walk by Amir and give a sideways glance into the reflective surface. I might stop a second and straighten my hair, wipe the mascara crumbs from under my eyes or pick the salad remnants from my teeth that my friends forgot to tell me about. It was a give and take relationship. Amir gave me a way to primp and prep, and I Windexed him, keeping him dust and toothpaste-splatter free. When I was going through chemo that relationship turned cloudy. I would dart past him and not peer at the reflective image. I didn't like what he was showing me, namely a blatant reminder that I was battling cancer. A fuzzy head, pale skin and weight gain all wrapped into one image that I believed wasn't the real me. What was it about that image that made the relationship so cloudy? *Ah,* I thought.... *I never defined myself as a cancer patient.* So Amir's depiction of me wrestled with my inner self. I was still enjoying and living life with my protection of denial. Except this reflection was a knife that cut away that denial to reveal the reality of my battle.

When my initial treatment was over, I began the process of rebuilding the relationship with Amir. I was able to stand in front of him and apply makeup. I could brush what was a large tuft of curly strands. The reflective image though is different. I have permanently changed. I am emotionally and mentally more mature. When I look at the reflection I see the change. So our relationship is being rebuilt one glance at a time. I am stronger, and as I continue to battle my cancer alien invasion, my applied cosmetics are war paint.

Ode to a Ponytail

When I was a child I had one of those Barbie heads with the hair that you could style. I remember trimming the hair with blunt safety scissors, knowing that it would greatly improve the look of Barbie staring back at me. When the cut was finished and I had thoroughly applied sky blue eye shadow to the plastic diva, I noticed the hair-cut was not very desirable. In fact, it resembled the time my mother had to cut bubble gum out of my hair when I accidentally fell asleep chewing. The cut was short, wispy, uneven and distorted.

I had just donned my first ponytail since chemo. It isn't long and flowing, but resembles that of a Sumo wrestler before he is about to step his jumbo sized body into the ring. I tugged and tugged to try to get all of the short wisps into a plastic holder. Success! I wore the Sumo ponytail all day.

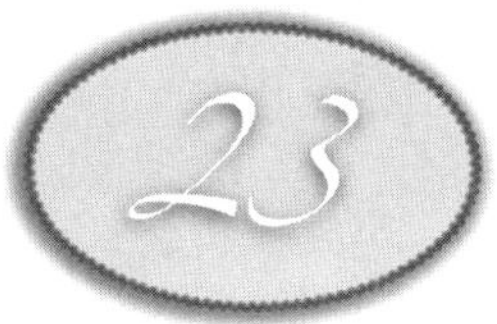

Attitude is Everything

GOING THROUGH THIS PROCESS MADE ME AWARE OF myself. I decided that there were two main reasons for keeping a good attitude. One is that it allowed me to maintain my sense of humor during my war, and two, I felt like if I had a bad attitude, no one was going to want to be around me. There were different ways I tried to accomplish this task. One was getting in touch with my inner rock star. Do you ever remember the times when you were younger and didn't have a care in the world? You felt great about how you looked and for the upcoming day. You were excited for the events and people you were going to meet. Well, I would go back to that place of joy and use my creativity and imagination to catapult me back to those times. This was a meditative state that switched my energy levels from bad to good in minutes. I shut the door on my past angers and failures and focused on trying to heal. This wasn't an easy process and it took practice. Just like learning to ride a bike. I would have to learn how to remind myself to move into a more positive mental attitude.

I also found that it was important to keep some semblance of status quo. Although tired and beat down from the treatment, there was something comforting in keeping my daily routines intact. Going to work and interacting with people became a therapy of distraction.

I found that my brain was always trying to move towards something that would totally take it over and quiet it in the moment. My acrylic painting did that for me, as I would only focus on the task at hand. The color, movement of my hand and focus of getting the layers just right kept me right in the present moment. Putting my energy toward my passion relieved my brain of the intense weight of the treatment. This activity lifted my mood and made it easier to cope with my increasing depletion of energy. A lot was taken from my body during treatment, but nobody could take my creativity.

Although many people asked me what I was going through and how I was doing I tried to stay on a more positive note than speak of the gory details. People who are not going through cancer usually are being polite and want to know how you are doing. They don't necessarily want to hear about the bad needle stick you got that day in chemo or the way that you felt nauseous most of the day. I found this out the hard way. When I first recounted a detailed play-by-play of some treatment incidents, a quick read of the non-veteran's face told me to switch gears. I saved those stories and notes for comrades in my survivor groups. This allowed me to keep my other relationships somewhat normal. Bringing up cancer consistently with others gave it a power I didn't like. It gave it an identity in which the past and future of it became more important than my present situation. My existence and presence in the here and now is what matters most. And lets face it, describing the details of a cancer war can scare the shit out of your friends and acquaintances.

Sex and Relationships

OF COURSE SEX IS ONE OF THE MOST IMPORTANT ACTS OF showing love. When you are going through treatment there isn't a lot to feel sexy about. I wanted to write about this candidly because it is a fact of life and I figure that Dr. Ruth had to have the talk with her mom about it at some point, so my mom reading this couldn't be too much of a shocker. Cancer creates a strain on relationships that is so severe that some relationships that were already having problems don't work. I first started dating my boyfriend three months before I was diagnosed. What a shit kicker. He was cute too. My boyfriend and I met online. I was immediately drawn to him by his wit and charisma. I had been out of a failed marriage for about a year and a half. I wasn't looking for love and was content living my life with two high maintenance Yellow Labradors. When I was diagnosed, I felt like Dorothy in the Wizard of Oz. I was caught in a tornado of confusion, and

Auntie Em was nowhere to be found. Only if I had those damn ruby slippers, I could just click myself away.

Besides family members, my boyfriend was one of the first people I confided in about my alien invasion. He sat quietly while I spilled my guts out about being diagnosed and what my future may or may not hold. There were so many unanswered questions. I was confused and not yet set on a course of action. I had to focus on me and my fight. The unknowns were so great that I questioned what my responsibility was in the relationship. After the shock of being diagnosed diminished, I decided that the best option would be to cut him loose. After all, he didn't sign up for this. So many thoughts were going through my head. Who would want to go through chemotherapy with a girlfriend that you just met? Who would want to go through the possibility of a girlfriend losing her breasts? I decided I would meet him for lunch and break the news to him. I wanted to give him a way out, but still let him leave with his dignity intact. My plan was to let him back out without it sounding like he would be a jerk for leaving his girlfriend during her time of need.

I decided talking with him during lunch would be as good a time as ever. We sat at the restaurant and I said, "I wanted to let you know that I feel like it is a good idea to take a break from our relationship. I feel like you didn't sign up for this and that maybe after eight months or so, if you are still interested we can pick up where we left off." After a long pause, he said, "Okay." I was prepared for that exact answer. I'm sure my face showed disappointment. I was pretty good at acting classes in school, but not Oscar material. He commanded a long pause before announcing, "Ha! I didn't think that is what you wanted…I was just testing you. I don't want to stop dating you…that's not what I want. I

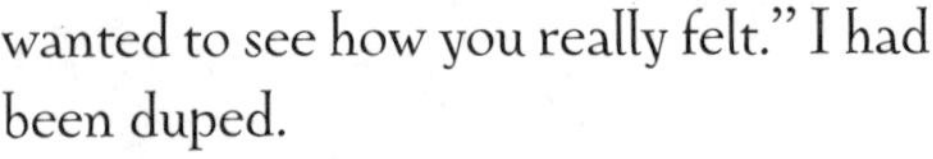

wanted to see how you really felt." I had been duped.

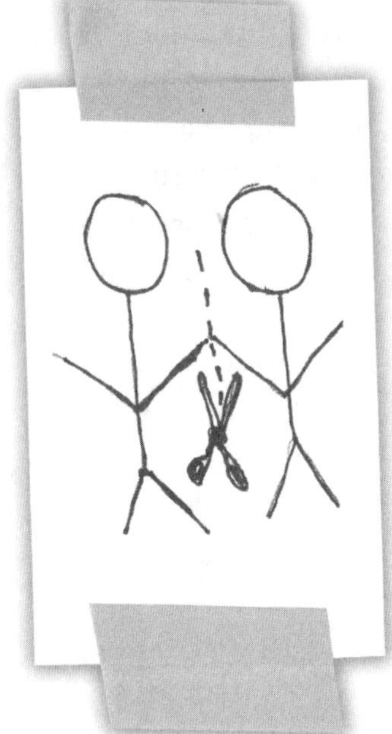

My boyfriend and I had sex almost every day when we were first dating. My married friends joked that we had some type of freak rabbit genes that caused us to cruise into sexual overdrive. I had never met anyone that I fit with so well emotionally and physically. All of these emotions would eventually lead to various strings of fears.

During my multiple surgeries I noticed that my sex life had tapered off. I had reserved myself to thinking that surgical drains and tubes sticking out of me surely can't be sexy. I became painfully aware that I wasn't getting any. No sex and not a lot of attention. I kept reading about all of these things you can do to make yourself feel sexy, including: buying new lingerie, perfume and getting a makeover. I started to believe "lights off" was the best remedy for a sexless relationship challenged by my cancer alien invasion.

As I started to get used to my new body, I realized more and more that successfully sexy was a strong state of mind. I had caught a short clip on a radio station announcing how to heighten your sex appeal. It included changing the way you make eye contact, keeping your shoulders back and increasing your intent listening skills to entice your potential partner. This seemed to make a lot more sense than just trying to alter my appearance. I started trading glances into the mirror for a peek into my confidence levels.

We started talking about the fact that I wasn't getting much attention and that I felt like he may not want me anymore. It concerned me that our sex life was like a tennis player wearing black at a Wimbledon tennis match: nowhere to be found.

It turns out that he thought sex would hurt me physically and he didn't want to take that chance. He wanted to protect me. Apparently, our communication had become about effective as two coffee cans with a string draped between them.

When Man's Role Changes from Hunter to Caregiver

THE MAN'S ROLE SIGNIFICANTLY CHANGES WHEN A WOMAN is going though breast cancer. For me, I was in the dating stage. My boyfriend was courting me, one of the most fun parts of starting a relationship. Cards left in unexpected places telling me how much he loved me. Surprise gifts. He was in hunter mode…and I was the target.

Lets face it, it's pretty darn flattering. All of these actions reiterate to our female selves that we are attractive, that we are wanted and desired, and that a man is going out of his way to get our attention. It's all part of the dance of courtship. When I was first diagnosed and I was dating, one of the reasons I wanted to cut my boyfriend loose was because I felt like his image of me as a vibrant young

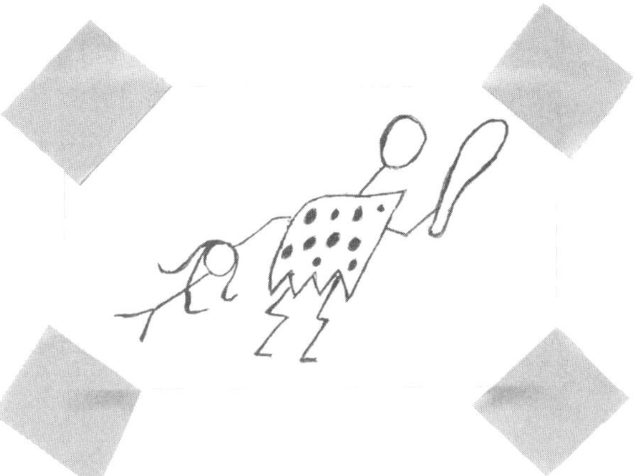

woman had been destroyed. All of these doubts sprang into my head about the courting process. Doubts about life and how it pertained to me. Would I still be desirable? Would I be ugly without hair? Would I become part of this secret club in which I would turn into an utter bitch cursing the world for my alien invasion?

I had a lot of pending questions. As we went through treatment, many of them began to unfold. The unfolding process wasn't neat and tidy like an American flag, more like a ship's sail wadded up and the jib slowly unfolding in the inconsistent breeze. Communication between my boyfriend and me became our constant ally. However, this is where feelings would really get trampled.

I think it started to go downhill for me when I started asking questions that I wasn't necessarily prepared for him to answer. For example, when I asked my boyfriend about our diminishing sex life and wanted to know if he still found me as attractive as ever... ..the answer wasn't a resounding, "yes". He explained to me that after my surgery he hadn't felt as attracted to my body as before. Again…I wasn't quite prepared for that. So I did what I do best when I am threatened…I retaliated. I cried, told him how shallow he was, and that if he couldn't handle it then maybe he should find someone else. The truth is…I had asked the question and was totally unprepared for the answer. So what was it I was looking for? A "No, honey, you don't look fat in that dress" kind of answer? After the upset emotions wore off, I thought about the answer that he had given me. At the risk of hurting my feelings he gave an honest answer, so I punished him. Not necessarily the best way to foster communication.

As treatments progressed, I was more tired than usual, and I wasn't in tip-top shape after surgery. My boyfriend was extremely aware of my pain. He was very gentle and caring, a far cry from his previous hunter persona. The pursuing faded away as he moved from hunter to protector and caregiver. Lack of communication started to creep in at this time, which did some damage to the relationship. I felt like I wasn't desirable. I wasn't wanted like the hunter once wanted me. To coin a very bad Italian movie phrase, "I was damaged goods." When we finally started verbally engaging in this topic, it turns out that I was way off the mark. In reality, he was trying not to hurt me, but to protect me from any type of pain. When we got over this speed bump, sexual activity resumed. Thank God. It was vital to share truthful concerns from both parties. This communication was crucial and promoted the emotional growth required to get through the rough parts. Communication, it turns out, would be the cornerstone of us moving through this situation. By recognizing the fear, resentment and anxiety, I was able to turn it down low enough to hear true concerns without the baggage of my past. Having preconceived notions of what someone should say as well as resentment and hurt feelings is one of the toughest self-discoveries. Once you are able to quell those feelings, you can have a dialog of truth that grows the relationship, not just banter designed to raise your own egocentric personal score.

My local support group of cancer survivors invited us to a member's house for a discussion about sex after breast cancer. There was a pretty good turn-out of ladies. The wine flowed as we sat down with a specialist in this field. We were all having the same issues. The camaraderie made it easier to ask difficult questions and the intimate setting at someone's house made the discussion more palatable and less like men's locker room talk. The room was void of men, which also made it more comfortable. We shared stories and problems, but most of all, we laughed.

Losing Significant Others

I WENT TO A FUNDRAISER FOR OUR YOUNG SURVIVORS GROUP recently. It was amazing. It was an art bra fundraiser to raise money for the young survivor group. Many survivors, artists and patrons had designed art bras to auction at the event. I was a gofer running around fielding questions and being an overall jack of all trades. I turned around and all of a sudden one of the survivors that I had not seen in a very long time walked in. I said, "Oh my God, I haven't seen you in forever! Where have you been?" Her answer was, "My husband left me. He said he couldn't handle it any longer." I couldn't believe it. Her husband walked out on her and their little girl.

As the night progressed, it was apparent that she was not the only one struggling with the Y-chromosome. Another young survivor friend confided in me that her boyfriend had been unfaithful. Again the reason was, "I just was having trouble handling it."

What is it about cancer that causes so many people that don't even have it to say they can't handle it? Fear has an ugly way of rearing its big old head. If our significant others were on the edge of a cliff slowly slipping over the edge with pebbles and rocks flying from underneath their feet, would we toss them a rope? The definitive answer is, "Yes!" Why are so many of us sliding and struggling with our diagnosis, yet so many fail to throw us a rope. In fact, it feels like some of us are kicked with a boot.

Many of us have gone through lumpectomies, sentinal node biopsies, mastectomies, radiation, chemotherapy, and so on. FEAR is our middle name. However, somewhere in that quagmire of medical merry-go-round, our fear grew weak, and we grew stronger. Why? Because we had to, we are needed. Needed by friends, family, children and colleagues. Maybe our strengths become intimidating. Maybe the change is so monumental that some no longer recognize us. Just maybe, we were intended for better situations.

I had a string of bad luck relationships before I was diagnosed. In fact, I was feeling a little jaded about the Y-chromosome in general. I wondered after being hurt if I would ever be able to love someone on that higher level. The level where you put someone before yourself. With the cancer diagnosis arriving after my divorce, I developed a bitter feeling about what the future might hold for my love life. I wondered if loving someone deeply would even be an option again. But I began to think about this loving concept. When you are really able to love someone on a very deep level, you become more vibrant. Your feelings, personality and experiences multiply. When or if you lose that person, you may experience a great pain. Sometimes that pain seems overwhelming, but the exponential growth obtained by that loving experience moves on with you through life. I decided I would have to make a choice. I would either choose to be bitter or choose to leave the bitterness behind to make room in my closet for happiness, spiritual growth and hot fudge sundaes.

Time

I REMEMBER THE FIRST ENCOUNTER I HAD WITH LEARNING how to tell time. My father had a plastic toy clock with hands that moved and caps that covered 5-minute, 10-minute, and 15-minute intervals. I was so preoccupied with the numbers that existed under the caps that I would completely forget about remembering what minute intervals were located where. On top of the forgetfulness, I felt the stress and impatience of my father looming over me. I could see his eyes bulging as I started pitching my incorrect guesses. Was this "quality time" spent with my father or toy time designed to create a short temper and unparalleled frustration?

I used to have a strange obsession with being on time. I know that it is the right thing to do. I know that it is the polite thing to do. My obsession was a fear that often made me a little neurotic. When I fly I have to double and triple check my tickets for the departure time. I'm not sure how this obsession started or whether it was a fear of people starting without me....or maybe being rude. I would check my watch several times before leaving the house, map out the exact route in my head and calculate anything I could think of that might make me late. I can't think of anything more finite than time.

Time is finite. I can't help but think that this is a big piece of my frustration with cancer. Cancer and time are not friends; they co-exist but play tug-o-war with each other. There is not a mud pit in the middle, just me balancing the rope's tension, the finite rope of time. Stretching and lengthening the line as far as I possibly can, I want time to win the blue ribbon while cancer loses its grip.

Gratitude

When I was going through my divorce, I felt like the whole world was falling apart. Being an overachiever, you aren't supposed to fail at anything. At the time, I started working with a wise mentor/lawyer designated to get me through this time unscathed. She talked about when you jump down into the ditch of unhappiness and despair it is often healthy to counteract these feelings with thoughts of gratitude.

I started trying this technique, especially when I felt so depressed that I felt ill. That weird stomach turning feeling that grips you below the belt. I was grateful for a wonderful family, my friends, my boyfriend and my two Yellow Labradors. Running through my mind, going over and over again what I was grateful for, pushed the fear, sadness, and pain down and lifted me up to rise above it.

When I was a teenager I used to complain about my appearance. "Mom, my legs are too short" or "I wish I had blonde hair." My mom had the swiftest way to dispel any thoughts of inadequacy. "At least you have legs," she would retort. I would look sideways at her raised eyebrows. Funny, that she could shut up my complaining with one brief utterance.

Gratitude is a powerful tool, lifting me up to a higher plain of happiness. Without it we would never be happy, always wanting more but never satisfied. Like when you are a kid at a birthday party and your best friend gets a bigger piece of chocolate cake. Its like climbing an endless ladder to get more stuff, and never really being happy with what we have now.

I realized that when I was first diagnosed, my "woe is me" attitude was not productive. Going into the chemo room and seeing all of the different people being treated, I realized that we were all in this together. I would often carry an object into the room and reach into my purse to look at it or feel it. Sometimes it was a piece of jewelry that reminded me of someone; sometimes it was a picture or card. It was purposely there to remind me of different things I was grateful for. I would periodically scroll through pictures in my phone. So many of them reminded me of what I held dear.

Self Rewards

After I was finished with my treatment schedule, I wanted to do something fun for me. So I went out and bought a metallic light blue convertible. Not really practical, it was just a two-seater with a lot of power. It was fun and that's what I was waiting for. I remember one time I was visiting the oncologist's office for a check up. I was riding down in the elevator and there was a mother and daughter in the elevator with me. The mother had been going through chemo treatments and her daughter was there to keep her company. I asked how they were doing and the daughter responded that her mother was going through a second round of chemo for cancer. I told them that I was a two-year veteran as well. As we left the elevator, I turned to the new shiny convertible that I had purchased after chemo. "This is what I bought myself after chemo," I exclaimed. She looked at me and said, "Good for you! I got something out of it too…a tummy tuck!" We both walked away laughing hysterically.

Rewarding myself was like hitting a milestone. I looked forward to every treatment that would end. It made a difference, like having that checkered flag being waved as you finish the race. Being a kid at heart allows you to look forward to those moments when you get your new toy or ice cream. It didn't really matter to me what the reward was, as long as I personally enjoyed it and I became even more grateful for the present moment.

Self-affirmations would become more important to me as I went through treatment. Taking care of myself and acting for my self preservation took front row in my personal theater. Developing strong networking and relationships allowed me to move through difficult times. Concentrating on reading books and Podcasts that uplifted me and kept my brain jogging became even more important. Relaxing and learning how to meditate gave my stress a vacation. Learning to relax my goal driven overachiever self became an integral theme. All of these elements were gifts to me. My criticism became a hitch-hiker and the love for myself a passenger.

Angels Are Amongst Us

I WOULD LIKE TO TALK ABOUT THOSE ANGELS AMONGST US that just with a comment, gesture or act of kindness make all the difference in the world to a person going through the cancer experience.

It was September, and my boyfriend and I decided to go to the small town of Gruene, TX. I was feeling a little tired, and I thought this small quaint German Texas town would be a good breath of fresh air and a nice change from the grind. I had very little hair at that point, more of a mange look, and I therefore donned a navy blue bandana to shield my head from the sun's rays. It was a beautiful day and the fresh air filled my lungs and helped me to relax.

There was a country fair going on. There were a number of vendors that were displaying their wares including jars of homemade preserves, jewelry, wood carvings, and much more. The town was

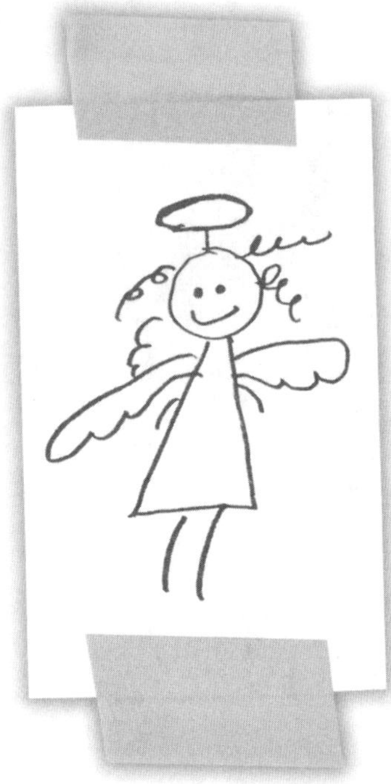

bustling with people. As I walked by I could feel people turn and stare at me, curious as to why I had no hair and sported a bandana. If I concentrated hard enough I felt like I had eyes in the back of my head watching the stares. I had tried to train myself to ignore these stares, but my training had failed. Then I started using my imagination to tell myself that I was famous. I was a rock star walking among the commoners.

As we got closer to the booths I noticed one woman selling homemade jewelry, nightlights and quilted items. I was picking up items off of her table and holding them up to the sunlight. She approached me and said, "Excuse me, I was just wondering if you were going through cancer treatments?" I told her that I was going through breast cancer treatments. She indicated that her daughter-in-law, who was in her thirties, had just undergone treatment for breast cancer and had gone through chemo as well. She held out her hand and inside her palm was a blue and silver angel pin. She blessed me and wished me the best of luck. I keep that pin on my dresser as a reminder of how one angel person can impact your life with one small gesture.

Another instance that sticks out in my mind was a rainy day after I had finished chemo. I decided that enough was enough with my wig. I had enough hair to at least look like a Marine soldier. I was dressed very girlie in a skirt, heels and a sweater and had applied plenty of make up. It was a good day. I had finished up chemo weeks before and was feeling a bit of energy in the air. I had just finished running in and out of the grocery store and I decided to leap over a puddle in the parking lot using my new-found energy. A pickup truck slowed down as I was walking to my car and the driver started to roll down the window. As he got closer I prepared myself to help this person with directions. This wasn't the case. There was a handsome older gentleman in the car with a very nice smile on his face. I asked, "Can I help you with directions?"

"Oh no," he replied. "I just wanted to tell you how great you look with that short hair." I laughed and said, "Well, six months of chemo gave me this hair, but I really appreciate you saying that."

He smiled and said, "You look amazing!" He proceeded to drive off and the rest of that day I had complete joy in my being.

I will continue to earn my angel wings by remembering and practicing what others have done for me. Believing in, supporting and empowering other patients, friends, family members and strangers has become one of my favorite activities. I personally like the element of surprise, when no one expects it. The impact is more enjoyable. It's amazing what can happen as those wings start to grow.

Candy-Coated Shell

AFTER ALL OF THE TREATMENTS WERE OVER, I WAS WORN out like last year's shoes. I felt ten years older. I looked in the mirror and wasn't quite sure who was looking back at me. I wondered if I would ever feel like my old self again. Nope. I had changed immensely. I have had different levels of transformation in my life. From young child to teenager, from teenager to adult, from adult to a spiritual self. Thinking about it, as a child I lived in the moment. I was only concerned about what was impacting me that day. A mere ride on a Big Wheel, enjoying an ice cream cone on a hot Texas day, punching my older brother's arm as I ran from the scene of the incident. There was no stress about bills, work or over thinking what I needed to accomplish in the future. I had not been imprinted yet with the worries of adulthood. Life was simple.

As I started to move into an older age bracket, all of the influences around me shaped me like silly putty. I was expected to get good grades. I was expected to achieve on a high level. I was expected to get a good job. My self and everyone around me watched as I grew into a more egocentric self. What do I have? What are my goals? What car will I drive? What clothes or jewelry will I own? Possessions and achievement existed on the top of my importance list. Looking back at those times, I am left wondering why the expectations of other people seemed so important.

After this life-altering event of cancer, I find myself returning to a more child-like state in that I once again am living in the moment. It feels like I read a significant book about my life and years later I read the same book and got a totally different, more mature message. My fundamental message is different. Years of swimming through a sea of depression, self doubt and cancer diagnosis have given me a ladder to climb up to the roof of a healthier self. The rat race style needed for achievement has subsided. I am no longer concerned with how people see me. The scar road maps all over my body are insignificant. What I own is insignificant. Who everyone wants me to be is insignificant. This road that I have navigated since my diagnosis has been bumpy with many speed bumps and potholes. Now, instead of focusing on the hardships in the road of life, I choose to focus on how much lighter my life is after dumping all of the personal heavy baggage I had been shouldering. My "self" has matured to incorporate a more complex chocolate inside and not just a candy-coated shell.

About the Author

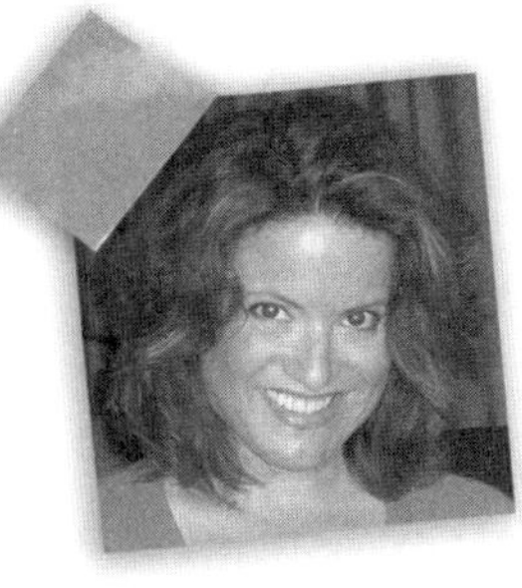

THE MOST IMPORTANT THING TO KNOW about Genae Girard is that she is who you have come to know her to be in these pages—and that she likes coffee ice cream. She enjoys the challenge and the thrill of 'belonging' in any environment, from motorcycle rally to a high-society gala fund raiser. And she has an amazing memory for recalling specific colors, which she uses frequently when choosing a paint color or designing computer graphics without the benefit of physical samples. Although these are the things that matter, there are distinctive life turning points to be appreciated about the journey of this first-time author.

As a self-proclaimed over-achieving type-A personality, Genae typically takes on monumental goals (remember—she likes challenge) and wins them. A native Texan, in 1994 at the young age of 26, Genae started a veterinary distributorship located in Central Texas. During her 13 years with the company, it was listed for three consecutive years in the Austin Business Journal's "50 Fastest Growing Private Companies," and #82 on the Inc. 500 list of "America's Fastest Growing Private Companies." In July 2006, that all changed when she got her diagnosis. This book is that story.

Three years later, she has now created a new corporation, www.ScreamingZebras.com, which focuses on reducing corporate stress, increasing personal productivity and supporting a vital corporate culture. She volunteers as a counselor for cancer survivors, is a patient advocate for self-education and taking personal control of treatment through a personalized plan (vs. the medical system dictating a 'fit-into-the-box' solution), and regularly participates in a local young survivors social group. Her humorous, real-world portrayal of getting through the trauma and recovery from breast cancer, as well as her zest as a patient advocate, has landed her the role of Stress Reduction Mentor and Speaker for many groups, organizations and events.

Genae is a plaintiff for the ACLU; together, they are fighting the U.S. patent office for granting one laboratory a patent on the breast cancer genes BRAC1 and BRAC2. She has been featured in numerous news programs, magazines, and radio shows such as: 60 Minutes, Wall Street Journal, New York Times, CBS News, USA Today and others.

A few more important things to know about Genae—she currently lives in Austin, Texas with her boyfriend, Bryant, and her two four-legged furry best friends. She often visits her horse, Blue, who helps cancer patients feel better through equine therapy. In her spare time, she maintains her passion for painting acrylics and donates many of her custom dog paintings to charities to raise funds for animal shelters (www.BowWowArt.com) and local breast cancer groups.